NOOM DIET COOKBOOK

A Comprehensive Beginners Guide to Noom Diet with 150+ Delicious Recipes to Improve Metabolism and Lose Weight Completely

EDWARD LINDA

Copyright © 2024 by Edward Linda

INTRODUCTION

The NOOM diet, more than just a conventional weight loss program, is a comprehensive approach that combines behavioral psychology, nutrition education, and personalized coaching to foster sustainable and healthy lifestyle changes. Rooted in the belief that lasting weight management involves addressing both physical and psychological aspects of eating, NOOM provides a unique and dynamic platform for individuals seeking a holistic approach to their well-being.

At the core of the NOOM philosophy is the understanding that successful weight loss and maintenance require a shift in mindset and habits. The program employs a color-coded system to categorize foods into green (low-calorie dense), yellow (medium-calorie dense), and red (high-calorie dense), guiding users toward making mindful and nutritious choices. This approach is not about restricting specific foods but rather encourages a balanced and colorful diet that supports overall health.

The psychology of eating takes center stage in NOOM, with a focus on addressing emotional triggers, establishing positive relationships with food, and fostering behavior change. By delving into the psychological aspects of nutrition, NOOM empowers individuals to identify and overcome obstacles, leading to long-term success in achieving and maintaining a healthy weight.

NOOM is not a one-size-fits-all solution; instead, it offers a personalized experience. Users set individualized goals, receive support from personal coaches, and engage with a vibrant community that shares experiences and encouragement. The incorporation of technology, such as the NOOM app, facilitates food logging, activity tracking, and access to a wealth of resources, making the journey towards a healthier lifestyle more accessible and interactive.

In essence, the NOOM diet transcends traditional weight loss programs, recognizing that lasting change requires a holistic approach that addresses both the body and mind. It empowers individuals to forge a positive relationship with food, make informed choices, and embark on a journey towards sustained well-being and a healthier life.

Understanding the NOOM Approach

The NOOM approach represents a revolutionary paradigm in the realm of weight management, combining behavioral psychology, nutrition education, and personalized coaching to create a holistic and sustainable strategy for achieving and maintaining a healthy weight. At its core, understanding the NOOM approach involves embracing a comprehensive lifestyle change that goes beyond mere dietary restrictions, focusing on the psychology of eating and long-term behavior modification.
• Behavioral Psychology:
• NOOM recognizes that successful weight management is intrinsically linked to behavior patterns and emotional triggers. By integrating principles of behavioral psychology, the program assists individuals in identifying

and reshaping unhealthy habits, addressing emotional eating, and fostering a positive mindset toward food.
• Color-Coded Food Classification:
• The NOOM approach employs a unique color-coded system that categorizes foods into green, yellow, and red. This system guides users toward making healthier choices by encouraging the consumption of nutrient-dense, low-calorie foods (green) and moderating the intake of medium-calorie (yellow) and high-calorie (red) foods. This approach emphasizes portion control and balanced nutrition rather than strict food elimination.
• Personalization and Goal Setting:
• Recognizing that each individual's journey is unique, NOOM offers a personalized experience. Users set individualized goals based on their preferences, health status, and aspirations. This tailored approach ensures that the program is adaptable to diverse lifestyles and promotes realistic and achievable objectives.
• NOOM App and Technology Integration:
• The NOOM app serves as a central hub, providing tools for food logging, physical activity tracking, and access to a vast repository of resources. The integration of technology enhances user engagement, making it easier to stay on track and fostering a sense of accountability.
• Coaching and Community Support:
• NOOM goes beyond the conventional self-help model by providing users with access to personal coaches who offer guidance, motivation, and support. Additionally, a vibrant community allows individuals to share experiences, challenges, and successes, creating a supportive network that enhances the overall journey.
• Education on Nutrition and Mindful Eating:

• Central to the NOOM approach is an emphasis on nutrition education. Users gain insights into making informed food choices, understanding nutritional values, and practicing mindful eating. This knowledge equips individuals with the tools to make sustainable and healthy dietary decisions.

The Science Behind NOOM

The science behind NOOM reflects a nuanced understanding of human behavior, cognitive processes, and nutritional principles. NOOM integrates evidence-based approaches to promote sustainable weight loss and overall well-being, acknowledging that successful health outcomes require a comprehensive understanding of the interplay between psychology and nutrition.
• Behavioral Psychology:
• Central to the NOOM approach is the incorporation of behavioral psychology principles. This involves recognizing and addressing the psychological factors that influence eating behaviors. NOOM helps users identify emotional triggers, unhealthy habits, and thought patterns related to food, fostering self-awareness and facilitating behavior change.
• Cognitive Behavioral Therapy (CBT) Techniques:
• NOOM draws from cognitive-behavioral therapy (CBT) techniques, a well-established therapeutic approach. CBT helps individuals identify and modify negative thought patterns and behaviors, promoting healthier decision-making and sustainable lifestyle changes.
• Color-Coding System:

• The unique color-coded food classification system used by NOOM is informed by nutritional science. Foods are categorized into green (low-calorie dense), yellow (medium-calorie dense), and red (high-calorie dense). This system helps users make informed choices by encouraging a higher intake of nutrient-dense, lower-calorie foods.
• Personalization and Goal Setting:
• NOOM's personalized approach is grounded in the principles of motivational psychology and goal-setting theories. Personalized goals are more likely to be achieved, and NOOM empowers users to set realistic and achievable objectives based on individual preferences, health status, and aspirations.
• Mobile App and Technology Integration:
• Leveraging technology, the NOOM app enhances user engagement and adherence. The app incorporates features such as food logging, activity tracking, and educational resources. This integration aligns with the principles of mobile health (mHealth), leveraging technology to improve health outcomes.
• Social Cognitive Theory:
• NOOM embraces social cognitive theory, emphasizing the role of observational learning and social support in behavior change. The inclusion of personal coaching and a supportive community aligns with this theory, providing users with positive role models and a network for encouragement and shared experiences.
• Motivational Interviewing:
• Motivational interviewing techniques are woven into the NOOM coaching model. This communication style aims to enhance motivation and facilitate behavior change by exploring and resolving ambivalence. Coaches employ

empathetic listening and collaborative goal-setting to empower users on their health journey.
• Nutrition Education:
• NOOM integrates evidence-based nutritional education to empower users with knowledge about healthy eating habits. Understanding nutritional values, portion control, and making informed choices contributes to sustained weight management.

The Psychology of Eating

The psychology of eating, a fundamental aspect of the NOOM approach, delves into the intricate relationship between emotions, behaviors, and food choices. This psychological perspective recognizes that our relationship with food is complex, extending beyond mere caloric intake to encompass emotional triggers, habitual patterns, and the social context of eating. Understanding the psychology of eating is pivotal in promoting mindful and sustainable changes in dietary behaviors. Here are key components of the psychology of eating within the NOOM framework:
• Emotional Eating Recognition:
• NOOM acknowledges that emotions often influence eating habits. Emotional eating, whether in response to stress, boredom, or joy, is addressed by fostering awareness. Users learn to identify emotional triggers and develop strategies to manage emotions without resorting to food.
• Mindful Eating Practices:

• Mindfulness, a core principle in the psychology of eating, involves being fully present and conscious during meals. NOOM encourages mindful eating practices, promoting a deeper connection with food, increased awareness of hunger and fullness cues, and a more satisfying eating experience.

• Behavior Change Strategies:

• NOOM employs evidence-based behavior change strategies rooted in cognitive-behavioral therapy (CBT). Users explore and modify automatic thought patterns related to food, challenging unhelpful beliefs and developing healthier responses to eating cues.

• Cognitive Restructuring:

• Cognitive restructuring, a key aspect of CBT, involves identifying and changing negative thought patterns associated with body image, self-worth, and food. NOOM guides individuals in challenging distorted beliefs, fostering a positive mindset, and cultivating healthier relationships with food.

• Self-Monitoring and Reflection:

• NOOM's emphasis on self-monitoring through the app facilitates ongoing reflection on eating behaviors. Users track their food intake, physical activity, and emotions, gaining insights into patterns and making informed decisions about their dietary choices.

• Positive Reinforcement:

• Positive reinforcement is woven into the NOOM coaching model, providing users with encouragement and celebrating small victories. This positive feedback loop enhances motivation and reinforces healthier eating habits.

• Individualized Approaches:

• Recognizing that individuals have unique psychological profiles and triggers, NOOM takes an individualized

approach to the psychology of eating. Personalized coaching and tailored goal-setting strategies consider each user's specific challenges and strengths.
• Social Support:
• The social aspect of eating is acknowledged by NOOM. The program incorporates a supportive community where users can connect, share experiences, and receive encouragement. Social support plays a vital role in sustaining positive changes in eating behavior.
By addressing the psychology of eating, NOOM empowers individuals to break free from restrictive dieting approaches and develop a healthier relationship with food. The program recognizes that lasting changes involve understanding and modifying the psychological factors that influence eating behaviors, fostering a positive and sustainable approach to weight management and overall well-being.

Personalized Meal Planning

Personalized meal planning is a cornerstone of the NOOM approach, reflecting the understanding that individual preferences, dietary requirements, and lifestyle factors play crucial roles in achieving and maintaining a healthy weight. This aspect of the NOOM program goes beyond generic meal templates, recognizing the importance of tailoring nutrition recommendations to the unique needs and goals of each user. Here's an exploration of the key elements of personalized meal planning within the NOOM framework:
• Individualized Goals:
• Personalized meal planning begins with the establishment of individualized goals. NOOM users set specific and

achievable objectives based on factors such as weight loss targets, health conditions, and preferences. These goals serve as the foundation for crafting a customized meal plan.

• Preferences and Dietary Restrictions:

• NOOM takes into account the diverse dietary preferences and restrictions of its users. Whether an individual follows a specific dietary pattern, has cultural considerations, or needs to accommodate allergies, the meal planning process is adapted accordingly.

• Nutrient-Dense Foods:

• The emphasis in personalized meal planning is on incorporating nutrient-dense foods. NOOM encourages the consumption of a variety of colorful fruits, vegetables, lean proteins, whole grains, and healthy fats to ensure that users receive a spectrum of essential nutrients.

• Flexible and Varied Choices:

• Personalized meal plans are designed to be flexible and varied. NOOM recognizes that monotony can hinder adherence to dietary recommendations, so the program encourages a diverse array of foods, flavors, and cooking methods to keep meals enjoyable and satisfying.

• Portion Control Guidance:

• NOOM integrates portion control guidance into personalized meal plans. Understanding appropriate portion sizes is crucial for achieving and maintaining a healthy weight. Users learn to recognize appropriate portions and avoid overeating.

• Balanced Macronutrients:

• The NOOM approach ensures a balance of macronutrients (carbohydrates, proteins, and fats) in each meal. This balance contributes to sustained energy levels, satiety, and overall nutritional adequacy.

• Meal Timing Considerations:

• Personalized meal plans also consider individual preferences regarding meal timing. NOOM recognizes that factors like meal frequency, timing, and the distribution of nutrients throughout the day can influence metabolism and adherence to the plan.

• Incorporation of Treats in Moderation:

• NOOM embraces the concept of moderation, allowing for the inclusion of treats or indulgences in a balanced and controlled manner. This approach avoids a restrictive mindset and encourages a healthy relationship with all types of food.

• Education on Smart Food Choices:

• The meal planning process involves education on making smart food choices. NOOM provides information on reading food labels, selecting nutrient-dense options, and making informed decisions when dining out or preparing meals at home.

• Continuous Adaptation:

• Personalized meal plans are not static; they evolve based on individual progress, preferences, and changing goals. NOOM's adaptability ensures that users can make adjustments to their meal plans as needed, fostering sustainability and long-term success.

Tailoring the Diet to Individual Preferences

Tailoring the diet to individual preferences is a key principle within the NOOM program, recognizing that adherence to a personalized and enjoyable eating plan is crucial for long-term success. This approach goes beyond traditional one-size-fits-all diets, acknowledging that individuals have unique tastes, cultural influences, and lifestyle considerations. Here's an exploration of how NOOM tailors the diet to individual preferences:

• Customized Goal Setting:

• NOOM starts by understanding each user's goals, whether they are focused on weight loss, improved health, or other objectives. The program then tailors dietary recommendations to align with these individual goals.

• Cultural Considerations:

• NOOM recognizes the impact of cultural influences on dietary preferences. Whether someone follows a specific cultural eating pattern or has specific culinary traditions, the program adapts recommendations to ensure compatibility with these preferences.

• Flexible Meal Choices:

• The NOOM approach encourages a wide variety of foods, allowing users to choose meals that align with their tastes. This flexibility helps prevent monotony and supports adherence to the dietary recommendations.

• Incorporating Favorite Foods:

• NOOM acknowledges that completely eliminating favorite foods can be unrealistic and may lead to feelings of deprivation. Instead, the program teaches users how to incorporate favorite foods in moderation while maintaining overall balance.

• Education on Smart Swaps:

• NOOM provides education on making smart food choices, including offering healthier alternatives to less nutritious options. This allows individuals to enjoy familiar flavors while making choices that align with their health goals.

• Guidance on Portion Control:

• Tailoring the diet involves providing guidance on portion control rather than strict food restrictions. This empowers individuals to enjoy the foods they love while managing overall caloric intake.

• Adapting to Dietary Preferences:

• Whether someone follows a vegetarian, vegan, or omnivorous diet, NOOM adapts its recommendations accordingly. The program respects and accommodates diverse dietary preferences, ensuring that users can adhere to their chosen eating style.

• Mindful Eating Practices:

• NOOM incorporates mindful eating practices, encouraging individuals to savor and enjoy their meals. This mindfulness allows users to connect with their food, enhancing the overall eating experience.

• Understanding Food Triggers:

• NOOM helps users understand their individual food triggers, whether related to emotions, stress, or specific situations. By recognizing these triggers, individuals can develop strategies to make mindful choices in response to them.

• Community Support:

• The NOOM community provides a platform for individuals to share their experiences and preferences. This supportive network allows users to exchange tips, recipes, and ideas, creating a sense of community around personalized dietary choices.

Adapting NOOM Principles to Different Dietary Preferences

Adapting NOOM principles to different dietary preferences is a fundamental aspect of the program, recognizing that individuals follow diverse eating styles based on cultural, ethical, or personal choices. The flexibility of NOOM allows users to incorporate its core principles while adhering to their preferred dietary patterns. Here's how NOOM can be adapted to various dietary preferences:

• Vegetarian and Vegan Diets:

• For individuals following vegetarian or vegan diets, NOOM tailors recommendations to ensure adequate plant-based protein sources, a variety of colorful vegetables, and plant-based fats. The program educates users on protein-rich plant foods, iron sources, and vitamin B12 supplementation if needed.

• Mediterranean Diet:

• NOOM principles align well with the Mediterranean diet, emphasizing whole grains, fruits, vegetables, lean proteins, and healthy fats. The program encourages the consumption of olive oil, nuts, and fish while promoting portion control and mindful eating practices.

• Low-Carb or Keto Diets:

• For those who prefer low-carb or keto diets, NOOM can be adapted by focusing on non-starchy vegetables, lean proteins, and healthy fats. The program provides guidance on carb-conscious choices while emphasizing the importance of nutrient density.

• Paleolithic (Paleo) Diet:

• NOOM can accommodate a Paleo-style diet by emphasizing lean meats, fish, fruits, vegetables, nuts, and seeds. The program supports individuals in making choices that align with the principles of the Paleo diet while maintaining overall nutritional balance.

• Flexitarian Approach:

• NOOM is well-suited for a flexitarian approach, allowing users to incorporate a variety of plant-based and animal-based foods. The program supports flexibility in dietary choices, promoting a balanced and mindful approach to eating.

• Gluten-Free Diet:

• NOOM accommodates gluten-free preferences by guiding users towards naturally gluten-free foods like fruits, vegetables, lean proteins, and gluten-free whole grains. The program educates on label reading and making informed choices within a gluten-free lifestyle.

• Cultural and Ethnic Considerations:

• NOOM respects cultural and ethnic dietary preferences. Whether someone follows a specific cultural eating pattern or has unique culinary traditions, the program adapts recommendations to honor these preferences while promoting a balanced diet.

• Intermittent Fasting:

• For individuals incorporating intermittent fasting, NOOM offers support by providing guidance on meal timing and balancing nutrient intake during eating windows. The program encourages users to make nutritious choices within the framework of their fasting schedule.

• Food Allergies or Sensitivities:

• NOOM takes into account food allergies or sensitivities, providing guidance on alternative choices and substitutions.

The program helps individuals navigate their dietary preferences while ensuring nutritional adequacy.

• Mindful and Intuitive Eating:

• NOOM principles align with mindful and intuitive eating practices. The program encourages individuals to listen to their body's hunger and fullness cues, fostering a positive relationship with food and promoting a sustainable approach to eating.

NOOM Food Logging

NOOM's food logging feature is a central component of the program, empowering users to track their dietary choices and gain insights into their eating habits. This tool is accessible through the NOOM app and serves as a dynamic platform for self-monitoring, fostering mindfulness, and facilitating personalized coaching. Here's an overview of how NOOM food logging works:

• User-Friendly Interface:

• The NOOM app provides a user-friendly interface for food logging, making it accessible and intuitive for users of various tech proficiency levels. The app is available on mobile devices, allowing users to log their meals anytime, anywhere.

• Extensive Food Database:

• NOOM features an extensive food database that includes a wide variety of foods and beverages. Users can search for specific items, scan barcodes, or manually enter nutritional information to log their meals accurately.

• Color-Coded System:

• The NOOM color-coded system is integrated into the food logging process. Users classify their meals into green (low-calorie dense), yellow (medium-calorie dense), and red (high-calorie dense) categories. This helps users visualize the nutritional composition of their diet at a glance.

• Meal and Snack Logging:

• Users log not only main meals but also snacks and beverages throughout the day. This comprehensive approach enables a holistic view of daily dietary patterns, aiding in identifying areas for improvement and celebrating successes.

• Portion Control Guidance:

• NOOM provides guidance on portion control within the food logging feature. Users learn to estimate and log portion sizes accurately, contributing to a better understanding of their caloric intake and overall nutritional balance.

• Nutrient Tracking:

• Beyond calorie counting, NOOM's food logging tracks various nutrients, including macronutrients (carbohydrates, proteins, and fats), fiber, and other essential vitamins and minerals. This detailed tracking enhances users' awareness of their nutritional intake.

• Personalized Coaching Insights:

• The data from food logging contributes to personalized coaching insights. Coaches can review users' logs, identify patterns, and offer tailored guidance and feedback based on individual progress and challenges.

• Integration with Other Features:

• Food logging is seamlessly integrated with other features of the NOOM app, such as physical activity tracking and goal setting. This integration allows users to have a comprehensive view of their health-related behaviors and goals in one place.

• Real-Time Feedback:
• Users receive real-time feedback as they log their meals. The color-coded system provides immediate insights into the nutritional quality of each meal, empowering users to make informed choices on the spot.
• Educational Resources:
• NOOM's food logging feature is complemented by educational resources. Users receive information on making healthier food choices, understanding nutritional labels, and developing sustainable eating habits.

Tracking Nutritional Intake

Tracking nutritional intake is a fundamental aspect of health management, and it plays a crucial role in the NOOM program. Here's an overview of how NOOM approaches the tracking of nutritional intake:
• Comprehensive Nutrient Tracking:
• NOOM goes beyond basic calorie counting by offering comprehensive nutrient tracking. Users monitor their intake of macronutrients (carbohydrates, proteins, and fats), micronutrients, fiber, and other essential components of a balanced diet.
• Food Database and Barcode Scanner:
• The NOOM app features an extensive food database, allowing users to search for a wide variety of foods. Additionally, the barcode scanner enables quick and accurate logging of packaged food items. This functionality streamlines the tracking process, making it more convenient.
• NOOM Color-Coded System:

• NOOM employs a color-coded system to categorize foods into green, yellow, and red, based on their caloric density and nutritional content. This visual representation aids users in making healthier choices and understanding the overall nutritional balance of their diet.
• Educational Insights:
• As users log their meals, NOOM provides educational insights into the nutritional content of foods. This information helps users become more informed about their dietary choices and fosters a better understanding of the impact of different foods on their overall health.
• Portion Control Guidance:
• NOOM emphasizes portion control as a key component of nutritional tracking. Users learn to recognize appropriate portion sizes, promoting a balanced and mindful approach to eating.
• Meal Timing Considerations:
• In addition to tracking what is eaten, NOOM encourages users to consider when they eat. Understanding meal timing and distribution of nutrients throughout the day can play a role in optimizing energy levels and supporting overall health.
• Feedback and Coaching:
• The nutritional tracking data contributes to the feedback and coaching provided by NOOM. Personalized coaching insights help users identify patterns, address challenges, and receive guidance on making healthier food choices based on their individual nutritional needs.
• Integration with Physical Activity:
• NOOM integrates nutritional tracking with physical activity monitoring. This holistic approach allows users to see the relationship between their dietary choices and their

energy expenditure, promoting a balanced and active lifestyle.

• User-Friendly Interface:

• The NOOM app offers a user-friendly interface for tracking nutritional intake. The intuitive design and accessibility make it easier for users to log their meals, snacks, and beverages, fostering consistent tracking habits.

• Encouragement of Mindful Eating:

• Beyond the numerical data, NOOM encourages mindful eating practices. Users learn to pay attention to hunger and fullness cues, fostering a healthier relationship with food beyond the quantitative aspects of tracking.

By combining technology, education, and behavioral insights, NOOM's approach to tracking nutritional intake is designed to be informative, empowering, and conducive to long-term health and well-being. The program aims to help users develop sustainable and mindful eating habits that align with their individual nutritional needs and goals.

NOOM and Exercise

NOOM recognizes the importance of regular physical activity as a crucial component of overall health and well-being. The program integrates features to encourage and support users in adopting and maintaining an active lifestyle. Here's an overview of how NOOM incorporates exercise into its approach:

• Personalized Activity Goals:

• NOOM starts by helping users set personalized activity goals based on their fitness levels, preferences, and health objectives. These goals are tailored to be realistic and achievable, promoting gradual progress.

• Activity Tracking:

• The NOOM app includes a feature for tracking physical activity. Users can log various types of exercises, including cardio, strength training, and flexibility exercises. This tracking provides a comprehensive view of their fitness routine.

• Integration with Wearables:

• NOOM seamlessly integrates with popular fitness wearables and devices. This integration allows users to sync their activity data, providing real-time updates on steps taken, calories burned, and other relevant metrics. This feature enhances accuracy and convenience.

• Educational Resources:

• NOOM offers educational resources on the benefits of regular exercise, different types of physical activities, and how to incorporate movement into daily life. This information empowers users to make informed choices regarding their fitness routines.

• Progress Monitoring:

• Users can monitor their progress over time through the NOOM app. The program provides insights into achievements, milestones, and improvements in physical fitness. This feedback reinforces positive behavior and encourages continued engagement.

• Coaching Support:

• NOOM's coaching model extends to physical activity. Personal coaches offer guidance and support related to users' exercise goals. Coaches may provide tips on workout routines, overcoming barriers to exercise, and maintaining motivation.

• Behavioral Strategies:

• NOOM incorporates behavioral strategies to promote consistent exercise habits. Users learn techniques for overcoming barriers, building routines, and developing a positive mindset toward physical activity. These strategies contribute to sustained engagement.

• Flexible Approach:

• Recognizing that individuals have varied preferences and fitness levels, NOOM adopts a flexible approach to exercise. Users can choose activities they enjoy, whether it's walking, running, cycling, or engaging in group fitness classes. This flexibility enhances adherence.

• Emphasis on Everyday Movement:

• NOOM encourages not only structured workouts but also everyday movement. Tips and strategies are provided to incorporate more activity into daily routines, such as taking the stairs, walking meetings, or stretching breaks.

• Community Support:

• The NOOM community serves as a supportive network where users can share their exercise experiences, challenges, and successes. This sense of community fosters motivation and a shared commitment to an active lifestyle.

The Role of Physical Activity in NOOM

Physical activity plays a pivotal role in the NOOM program, contributing to the holistic approach to health and wellness. Here's an in-depth look at the role of physical activity in NOOM:

• Goal Setting:

• NOOM starts by helping users set personalized physical activity goals based on their individual fitness levels, preferences, and health objectives. These goals are designed to be achievable and align with overall wellness targets.

• Activity Tracking:

• The NOOM app includes a robust activity tracking feature. Users can log various types of exercises, monitor their daily steps, and record workouts. This tracking provides users with a clear overview of their physical activity patterns and progress.

• Integration with Wearables:

• NOOM seamlessly integrates with popular fitness wearables and devices. This integration allows users to sync data, such as steps taken, calories burned, and heart rate, providing real-time insights into their overall activity levels.

• Personalized Coaching Support:

• NOOM's coaching model extends to physical activity, with personal coaches offering guidance and support related to users' exercise goals. Coaches provide motivation, share tips on effective workouts, and address challenges users may encounter in maintaining an active lifestyle.

• Educational Resources:

• NOOM provides educational resources on the importance of regular exercise for physical and mental well-being. Users gain insights into the health benefits of different types of activities and learn how to incorporate movement into their daily lives.

• Behavioral Strategies:

• Behavioral strategies are woven into NOOM's approach to physical activity. Users learn techniques for building sustainable exercise habits, overcoming barriers, and cultivating a positive mindset toward fitness. These strategies contribute to long-term adherence.

• Flexible Exercise Choices:

• NOOM acknowledges that individuals have diverse preferences when it comes to physical activity. The program encourages users to choose activities they enjoy, whether it's walking, cycling, swimming, or engaging in group fitness classes. This flexibility promotes adherence.

• Progress Monitoring:

• Users can monitor their progress over time through the NOOM app. The program provides feedback on achievements, milestones, and improvements in physical fitness. This progress tracking serves as a motivational tool for users to stay committed to their goals.

• Everyday Movement Emphasis:

• NOOM emphasizes the importance of everyday movement. In addition to structured workouts, users receive tips on incorporating more activity into their daily routines, such as taking breaks to stretch, opting for active commuting, or participating in recreational activities.

• Community Engagement:

• The NOOM community serves as a platform for users to share their physical activity experiences, exchange tips, and provide mutual support. This sense of community fosters a collective commitment to leading an active and healthy lifestyle.

NOOM and Weight Loss

NOOM is widely recognized for its effectiveness in supporting weight loss through a comprehensive and personalized approach. Here's an overview of how NOOM addresses weight loss:

• Behavioral Change Focus:

• NOOM distinguishes itself by prioritizing behavioral change as a fundamental aspect of weight loss. The program acknowledges that sustainable results are achieved through modifying habits, fostering a positive mindset, and addressing the psychological aspects of eating.

• Individualized Goal Setting:

• NOOM helps users set individualized and realistic weight loss goals. These goals take into account factors such as starting weight, target weight, health considerations, and the pace of progress. This personalized approach enhances the likelihood of achieving and maintaining weight loss.

• Nutritional Guidance:

• NOOM provides guidance on creating a balanced and nutritious diet through its color-coded system. Users learn to categorize foods into green, yellow, and red, helping them make informed choices that contribute to a calorie deficit, a key factor in weight loss.

• Food Logging and Accountability:

• The NOOM app features a food logging component that encourages users to track their meals and snacks. This practice promotes mindfulness, accountability, and a better understanding of eating habits, facilitating weight loss progress.

• Education on Smart Food Choices:

• NOOM offers educational resources on making smart food choices, understanding nutritional labels, and practicing portion control. This knowledge empowers users to make informed decisions that align with their weight loss goals.

• Regular Physical Activity:

• Physical activity is integrated into the NOOM approach as a crucial component of weight loss. The program helps users set and track personalized activity goals, promoting an active lifestyle that contributes to overall calorie expenditure.

• Behavioral Strategies for Long-Term Success:

• NOOM focuses on equipping users with behavioral strategies for long-term success. This includes addressing emotional eating, recognizing triggers, and building sustainable habits that extend beyond the initial weight loss phase.

• Coaching Support:

• Personalized coaching is a key feature of NOOM, providing users with support, motivation, and guidance throughout their weight loss journey. Coaches offer insights, celebrate successes, and assist users in overcoming challenges.

• Community Engagement:

• The NOOM community serves as a platform for users to connect, share experiences, and provide mutual support. This sense of community contributes to motivation and accountability, enhancing the overall weight loss experience.

• Holistic Well-Being:

• NOOM promotes a holistic approach to well-being, recognizing that weight loss is interconnected with mental and emotional health. The program encourages users to cultivate a positive relationship with food, body image, and self-esteem.

Success Stories and Testimonials

NOOM has garnered numerous success stories and testimonials from individuals who have experienced positive transformations in their health and well-being. These testimonials highlight the effectiveness of NOOM's personalized approach to weight loss and overall wellness. While I can't provide specific testimonials, I can offer a general sense of the types of success stories associated with NOOM.

• Sustainable Weight Loss:

• Users often share stories of achieving and maintaining their weight loss goals with NOOM. These success stories emphasize the program's focus on sustainable behavior change and the adoption of healthier habits.

• Improved Relationship with Food:

• Many testimonials highlight how NOOM has helped individuals develop a healthier and more positive relationship with food. Users often mention overcoming emotional eating, making smarter food choices, and learning portion control.

• Increased Physical Activity:

• Success stories often include anecdotes about individuals incorporating more physical activity into their lives. NOOM's personalized activity goals and tracking features contribute to success in adopting a more active lifestyle.

• Enhanced Mental Well-Being:

• Some users attribute improvements in mental well-being to their experience with NOOM. Success stories may discuss increased confidence, better self-esteem, and a more positive mindset toward overall health.

• Community Support and Motivation:

• Testimonials frequently highlight the value of community support within the NOOM platform. Users appreciate the motivation and encouragement they receive from coaches and fellow community members, contributing to their success.

• Education and Awareness:

• Success stories often emphasize the educational aspect of NOOM, with users expressing newfound awareness of nutritional choices, understanding of their eating habits, and knowledge about creating a balanced lifestyle.

• Long-Term Lifestyle Changes:

• Many individuals share how NOOM has empowered them to make long-term lifestyle changes. Success stories often focus on the sustainability of the program's approach and the continued positive impact on users' health and well-being.

• Positive Coaching Experiences:

• Testimonials may highlight positive interactions with NOOM coaches. Users often appreciate the personalized guidance, insights, and motivation provided by coaches throughout their journey.

It's important to note that individual experiences with NOOM can vary, and success is influenced by factors such as commitment, adherence to the program, and individual circumstances. For more specific success stories and testimonials, individuals interested in NOOM may explore the program's official website or community forums where users often share their experiences.

Nam Phrig Noom (Northern Thai Pounded Roasted Chili Dip) Recipe

Ingredients
• 4 large hot green chiles, such as Anaheim or Chinese long green capsicum
• 4 whole very small shallots (about 1 inch in diameter), unpeeled (see note)
• 5 medium cloves garlic, unpeeled
• 2 tablespoons Thai shrimp paste or fish sauce
• 1/3 cup roughly chopped cilantro, including the stems
• Kosher salt
• 2 teaspoons juice from 1 lime
• Boiled eggs, sliced cucumbers, fried pork rinds, steamed green or long beans, and/or steamed pumpkin to serve

Directions
• Preheat a broiler to high heat and adjust rack to 3 inches below heating element. The goal is to get it as close as possible while still allowing a cast iron skillet to be placed underneath. Preheat cast iron skillet on a burner over high heat until lightly smoking, about 5 minutes.
• Place chilies, shallots, and garlic in skillet and place under the broiler. Broil, turning vegetables every few minutes, until darkly charred on all surfaces, about 10 minutes total. Some vegetables may cook faster than others; remove each vegetable as it cooks and transfer to a medium bowl. When

all vegetables are cooked, cover bowl tightly with foil and allow to steam for 10 minutes.

• If using shrimp paste, smear shrimp paste on a piece of heavy-duty aluminum foil. Place under the broiler and broil until aromatic, about 30 seconds. Remove from oven and set aside. (If using fish sauce, skip to next step.)

• Carefully peel chilies, garlic, and shallots and discard skins. Transfer to a large mortar and pestle. Add cilantro leaves and stems and shrimp paste (if using fish sauce, do not add until next step). Add a heavy pinch of salt. Pound until a rough, spoonable paste is formed, about 5 minutes.

• Stir in lime juice and fish sauce (if using). Season to taste with more salt if desired. Serve with steamed or raw vegetables, boiled eggs, and fried pork rinds. Leftover nam phrig noom can be stored in an airtight container in the refrigerator for up to 1 week.

Low-Calorie Mushroom Soup

EQUIPMENT
• Kitchen knife
• 6-8 quart pot

INGREDIENTS
• 1 tbsp olive oil extra virgin
• 1 tbsp butter (optional)
• 1 onion large (or 2 medium)
• 24 oz white mushrooms
• 24 oz any other type of mushrooms
• 8 cups chicken broth low sodium

- 8 cups vegetable broth
- 2 cups water
- 2-4 stems thyme fresh
- 1-4 bay leaves
- 1 cup wild rice (or wild rice blend) dry
- salt and pepper to taste

INSTRUCTIONS
- Heat a large pot and add the olive oil and butter (omit butter to keep recipe to 75 caloires/cup)
- Dice onion and sauté in the oil on medium heat until soft, stirring frequently
- Add sliced mushrooms, thyme, bay leaves, salt and pepper to the pot. Sauté and stir on medium heat until soft (10-15 minutes).
- Add broth and water to pot and increase heat.
- Bring to a boil, then reduce heat and simmer for at least 20 minutes
- Remove thyme stems and bay leaves.
- Bring back to boiling and add dry rice. Reduce heat and simmer according to the package instructions on the rice (about 45 minutes).

NOTES
1. We serve this soup warm with a side of sliced apples, salad, or even a toasted English muffin topped with shredded parmesan cheese and Greek seasoning.
2. We love pepper and will add about a tablespoon when we cook this recipe.

Noom Friendly Instant Pot Brown Rice Chicken Risotto

Ingredients
- 2 cups water
- 2 tbsp olive oil
- 1 red onion
- 3 large carrots
- 1 large can of diced tomatoes in juice
- 1 1/4 cups brown rice
- To taste salt and pepper
- 3 frozen chicken thighs

Cooking Instructions
- Always remember to wash the rice. Chop up the onion and carrots. I tend to use baby carrots because that is what I have in the fridge for my kids. It isn't required that the chicken is frozen but it is certainly very convenient.
- Add water, olive oil, the vegetables, rice, salt, and pepper to the Instant Pot and stir. Then place the frozen chicken in the middle on top of the mixture.
- Cook on high pressure for 25 minutes and then let naturally cool. Pull the chicken, stir, and serve.

Instant Pot Mongolian Beef

INGREDIENTS
- 1–1/2 lb flank steak, sliced into 1/2" strips (~3–4 inches long)
- 1 Tbsp olive oil

- 1 red bell pepper, sliced thin
- 1 large carrot, peeled & sliced thin
- 1 red onion, sliced thin
- 3 cloves garlic, minced
- 1 tsp fresh ginger, minced
- 3/4 cup tamari or soy sauce
- 1/3 cup brown sugar
- 1/3 cup + 2 Tbsp water
- 2 oz. orange juice
- 2 Tbsp cornstarch
- Red pepper flakes, optional
- Green onion, sliced thin, optional

INSTRUCTIONS

1. Place all ingredients except 2 Tbsp water and cornstarch in a pressure cooker (I used Instant Pot), stir well to combine.

2. Close pot (make sure vent is closed) and cook on manual mode for 8 minutes.

3. Allow beef to cool in pot via natural pressure release for 10 minutes.

4. Open pot (may need to vent before opening), cancel manual and turn to Saute mode.

5. In a small bowl, whisk together 2 Tbsp water + 2 Tbsp cornstarch. Add to pot, stir and allow to cook for ~3-4 minutes to thicken.

6. Serve over rice, top with red pepper flakes & green onions if desired & enjoy!

NOTES

1. Slow Cooker Directions: Follow the same directions, cook on low for 6-8 hours and then add in cornstarch/water mixture

Chicken Salad With Fennel - Noom

INGREDIENTS
• 354 grams Boneless chicken breasts ; shredded
• 1/4 cup Greek nonfat yogurt
• 28 grams Mayonnaise
• 2 tablespoons Parmesan grated
• 1 gram lemon zest
• 2 tablespoon lemon juice
• 1/2 bulb fennel ; chopped
• 3 gram Green onions ; chopped
• 3 grams Fresh basil

INSTRUCTIONS
1. Mix all ingredients together (131 calories p/serving)

Easy and healthy Nigerian Jollof rice recipe

Ingredients
1. 500 grams Long grain rice
2. 500 ml Vegetable Stock The two amounts of vegetable stock are used separately
3. 750 ml Vegetable Stock The two amounts of vegetable stock are used separately
4. 400 grams can Peeled plum tomatoes
5. 4 Red bell peppers (deseeded and cut into chunks)
6. 1 medium Red onion (thinly sliced) Keep onions separately as used at different points
7. 2 medium Red onions (roughly chopped) Keep onions separately as used at different points

8. 1 Scotch Bonnet chilli pepper Deseeded if preferred. If you like very spicy then add two here!

9. 3 tbsp Tomato Puree

10. 2 tsp Jollof Seasoning (made in bulk with 1.5 tbsp onion granules, 0.5tbsp mixed spice, 0.5tbsp dried thyme, 0.5tbsp ground black pepper, 0.5tsp cinnamon, 0.5tsp cayenne pepper, 0.5tsp garlic granules, large pinch of salt) alternatively use jerk seasoning for ease.

11. 1.5 tsp Dried Thyme

12. 2 Dried bay leaves

13. Low-Calorie Cooking Spray

Instructions

1. Using a jug blender, combine the tinned tomatoes and their juice, red bell peppers, chopped onions (NOT the sliced ones!) and the chilli pepper until smooth then set aside.

2. In a large lidded saucepan add the rice and 500ml of stock and bring to the boil. Reduce heat and allow to cook for around 5 minutes with the lid on until the water is absorbed by the rice. Don't panic that the rice is not cooked at this stage, it is not supposed to be.

3. Meanwhile, spray a large lidded wok or frying pan well with low-calorie cooking spray and place over medium heat.

4. Fry sliced onion for 2 minutes then add tomato puree, Jollof seasoning, dried thyme and bay leaves and fry for a further 2 minutes.

5. Add the blended chilli, tomato and onion mix to the pan and cook on a medium heat for 10-12 minutes. This allows the tomatoes to cook and the onions may sting your eyes a little at this point!

6. Add 500ml of stock to the pan along with the parboiled rice, stir and cover the pot with a lid. Turn the heat down to low and cook for 15 minutes.

7. Remove lid and stir well to ensure it is not sticking then add a further 250ml of stock and replace the lid. Cook for a further 15 minutes. stirring every 5-10 minutes to prevent it sticking.

8. If you feel the rice is too hard, add an extra 150ml of stock at this point and allow to absorb then remove from heat.

9. Remove the lid and cover with a clean tea towel. Leave to stand for 30 minutes.

10. Serve and enjoy! I served mine with some chunks of fresh tomatoes but you can serve however you wish.

Notes

1. If you prefer the Jollof to have a smokier taste, as they call party rice in west Africa, then this is easily done. Before removing from the heat at the end turn up the heat to full and allow to burn and crackle on the bottom of the pan for 3-5 minutes. Leave the lid on to stand for 30 minutes. this gives the smokier tasty of the classic Nigerian Party rice.

Noom Friendly Instant Pot Green Bean Jambalaya

Ingredients
• 4 links cooked chicken sausage sliced
• 2 cups uncooked brown rice washed
• 1 can diced tomatoes
• 1 cup chopped green beans

- 1 diced celery heart
- 1 diced onion
- 6 tbsp minced garlic
- 2 tbsp cumin
- 2 tbsp coriander
- 2 tbsp chili powder
- 1 tbsp paprika
- 1 tbsp thyme
- 1 tbsp pepper
- 1 tsp salt
- 4 packets chicken broth
- 2 cups frozen succotash vegetables (corn, edamame, pepper)
- 3 cups hot water
- 6 slices turkey bacon cut into chunks

Cooking Instructions
- Added all ingredients except for the bacon to the Instant Pot. Stir until the spices and vegetables have been mixed together.
- Lie the bacon on top of the mixture.
- Set the Instant Pot to cook for 30 minutes on soup mode. Natural cooling is optional. Using the quick release is perfectly fine.

Tuna Niçoise Salad

Ingredients
6–8 servings
¾ cup extra-virgin olive oil
¼ cup fresh lemon juice
2

Tbsp. Dijon mustard

1 tsp. honey

1 tsp. freshly ground black pepper

1 tsp. kosher salt, plus more

6 large eggs

1 lb. green beans, trimmed and/or new or baby potatoes, halved if larger

4 cups thinly sliced seedless cucumbers

3 cups oil-packed tuna

Olives, capers, peperoncini, pickles, anchovies, or other pickled-briny ingredients, drained well (for serving)

Flaky sea salt

Preparation

1. Whisk ¾ cup extra-virgin olive oil, ¼ cup fresh lemon juice, 2 Tbsp. Dijon mustard, 1 tsp. honey, 1 tsp. freshly ground black pepper, and 1 tsp. kosher salt in a medium bowl; set niçoise salad dressing aside.

2. Bring a medium pot of salted water to a boil. Carefully add 6 large eggs and cook 7 minutes. Using a slotted spoon, transfer eggs to a bowl of ice water (keep pot over high heat); chill eggs until cold, about 5 minutes. Peel; set aside.

3. Meanwhile, add 1 lb. green beans, trimmed and/or new or baby potatoes, halved if larger to the same pot of boiling water and cook until just tender, 2–4 minutes for green beans, 10–15 minutes for potatoes. Using a slotted spoon, transfer to bowl of ice water; let sit until cold, about 3 minutes. Transfer to paper towels; pat dry.

4. To serve, slice eggs in half and arrange on a large platter with green beans and/or potatoes, 4 cups seedless cucumbers, thinly sliced on a diagonal, and 3 cups oil-packed tuna. Top with olives, capers, peperoncini, pickles, anchovies, or other pickled-briny things, drained well,

sprinkle with flaky sea salt, and drizzle some reserved dressing over. Serve with remaining dressing alongside.

5. Do Ahead: Niçoise salad dressing can be made 5 days ahead; cover and chill. Eggs can be boiled and vegetables blanched 2 days ahead; cover and chill separately.

26 BEST NOOM DIET RECIPES

INGREDIENTS
- 1.   Avocado And Egg Noom Recipe
- 2.   Tropical Raspberry Smoothie
- 3.   30 Minute One Pan Chicken Fajitas
- 4.   Turkey Mince Chilli for Weight Loss
- 5.   Shrimp Biryani
- 6.   Pf Chang's Chicken Lettuce Wraps
- 7.   Low-Carb Greek Yogurt Broccoli Salad
- 8.   Roasted Vegetables
- 9.   Chicken Tortilla Soup
- 10.Key West Grilled Chicken
- 11.Roasted Butternut Squash Soup
- 12.Overnight Oats
- 13.1-Minute Instant Pot Quinoa with Veggies
- 14.Turkey Avocado Burgers
- 15.Mediterranean Pasta Salad
- 16.Baked Asparagus and Mushroom Pasta
- 17.Healthy Ground Turkey Lettuce Wraps
- 18.Cauliflower Shrimp Fried Rice
- 19.Sweet Potato Apple Sausage Skillet
- 20.Berry and Apple Crumble
- 21.Healthy Greek Yogurt Ranch Dressing
- 22.Crack Carrots {The Best Roasted Carrots}
- 23.High Volume Taco Meal Prep Bowls

• 24.Baked Shrimp Taquitos
• 25.Zucchini Bites Recipe
• 26.Egg Roll In A Bowl

INSTRUCTIONS
1. Choose your favorite recipe.
2. Click the link of your favorite recipe.
3. Follow the instructions of the linked recipe.
4. Enjoy!

Winter Squash Risotto

Ingredients
• 5 cups reduced-sodium chicken broth, or vegetable broth
• 2 tablespoons extra-virgin olive oil
• 3 medium shallots, thinly sliced
• 3 cups chopped peeled butternut, hubbard, red kuri or kabocha squash (1/2-inch pieces)
• 2 cups shiitake mushroom caps, thinly sliced
• ½ teaspoon dried thyme
• ½ teaspoon salt
• ¼ teaspoon freshly ground pepper
• 1/8 teaspoon crumbled saffron threads, (optional)
• 1 cup arborio rice
• 1/2 cup dry white wine, or dry vermouth
• ½ cup finely grated Parmigiano-Reggiano cheese

Directions
1. Place broth in a medium saucepan; bring to a simmer over medium-high heat. Reduce the heat so the broth remains steaming, but is not simmering.

2. Meanwhile, heat oil in a large saucepan over medium heat. Add shallots; cook, stirring, until fragrant, about 1 minute. Stir in squash and mushrooms; cook, stirring often, until the mushrooms give off their liquid, about 5 minutes. Add thyme, salt, pepper and saffron (if using); cook for 30 seconds. Add rice; stir until translucent, about 1 minute. Add wine (or vermouth) and cook, stirring, until almost absorbed by the rice, about 1 minute.

3. Stir in 1/2 cup of the hot broth; reduce heat to a gentle simmer and cook, stirring constantly, until the liquid has been absorbed. Continue adding the broth 1/2 cup at a time, stirring after each addition until all the liquid has been absorbed, until the rice is tender and creamy, 30 to 40 minutes total. (You may have some broth left.) Remove from the heat and stir in cheese.

Tips

1. Literally the dried stigma from Crocus sativus, saffron is the world's most expensive spice. Over 75,000 flowers are required for each pound of saffron. Fortunately, a little goes a long way. It's used sparingly to add golden yellow color and flavor to a wide variety of Middle Eastern, African and European-inspired foods. Find it in the specialty-herb section of large supermarkets, gourmet-food shops and tienda.com. Wrapped in foil and placed in a container with a tight-fitting lid, it will keep in a cool, dry place for several years.

Corn & Tomato Chowder

INGREDIENTS
• 1 tsp butter unsalted

- 1 cup chopped onions
- 1 cup chopped celery
- 3 cups boiled potatoes peeled, diced
- 1 bay leaf
- 2 cups chicken broth reduced-sodium
- 1 1/2 cups canned diced tomatoes with liquid
- 1 1/2 cups frozen corn thawed
- 1 1/2 cups milk nonfat
- black pepper freshly ground

INSTRUCTIONS

• Lightly spray a 4-5 quart non-stick pot with cooking spray. Add the butter and place over medium heat. Add the onions and cook, stirring, 5 minutes. Add the celery and potatoes and cook, stirring occasionally, for 2 minutes

• Add the bay leaf and broth and bring to a boil. Cover the pot and cook 20 minutes, stirring occasionally, for 2 minutes

• Remove the bay leaf, puree 2 cups in a blender or food processor, and return to the pot

• Stir in the tomatoes, corn, and milk. Return the soup to a simmer. Cover the pot and cook 20 minutes, stirring occasionally, for 2 minutes.

• Stir in a few grindings of the black pepper. Garnish with parsley.

NOTES

1. This tasty chowder recipe from Noom combines the flavors of tomato and corn. It's rich in texture yet light and healthy. Good to eat for lunch or to serve with dinner!

Low-Calorie Chicken Tortilla Soup

EQUIPMENT
• Large pot
• Kitchen knife
• Blender, immersion blender, potato masher, or fork

INGREDIENTS
• 1 tbsp olive oil extra virgin
• 2 large bell peppers any color
• 2 onions small
• 2 cloves garlic minced
• 6 cups chicken broth low sodium
• 4 cups water
• 2 cans Rotel tomatoes with habaneros 10 oz. cans
• 1 can diced green chiles 4 oz can
• 3 tbsp tomato paste
• 2 lbs. cooked chicken breast boiled and shredded OR browned and chopped
• 2 cans cannelloni beans 15 oz. cans (with liquid)
• 3 tsp cumin
• 2 tsp garlic powder
• Salt to taste
• 1 jalapeño pepper thinly sliced, for garnish
• Yellow corn tortillas

INSTRUCTIONS
• Heat a large pot and add olive oil.
• Dice bell peppers and onions and saute in the oil on medium heat until soft. Add minced garlic.
• Add chicken broth, water, Rotel, green chilis, and tomato paste to pot. Stir.

• Bring to a boil, then reduce heat and simmer for 30 minutes or so.
• Add cooked chicken breast, cumin, garlic powder, and salt to taste.
• Using a blender or immersion blender, puree one can of the cannelloni beans. If you don't have a blender, crush the beans using a masher or a fork until smooth.
• Simmer for 10 minutes, then add the can of whole cannelloni beans, and the pureed/smashed cannelloni beans.
• While soup is simmering, cut corn tortillas in small strips and spread them out on a cookie sheet. Spray with cooking spray, then sprinkle with cumin and chili powder (or taco seasoning) and bake at 375 degrees until golden brown and crispy.
• Serve soup with crisp tortilla strips and fresh jalapeño slices

NOTES

1. We've found that the can of pureed/smashed beans really gives the soup a creamy texture without adding cream (and the calories that come with it).

Nam Prik Noom (Thai Green Chilli Sauce)

Ingredients
• 3 medium heat or mild large green chillies
• 3 Thai green chillies
• 2 medium onions
• 10 cloves garlic
• 1 medium aubergine
• 1 large tomato
• 1 tsp palm sugar

• 2 Tbsp fish sauce
• 2 Tbsp lime juice
Garnish
• chopped chives, spring onions or fresh coriander
• strips of green chilli

Instructions
• Place the aubergine on a low open flame on the gas stove for 10 minutes, turning it around a couple of times.
• Get all the other ingredients ready in the meantime. Top the onions & garlic as mentioned above, that is, slice the non pointy ends off.
• When the aubergines has had it time, place everything under a medium grill (halfway) for about 10 minutes, turning once. You'll find the little chillies going completely soft first, take them out if you prefer, but I like the "overdone" flavour, it's sweet.
• Place everything apart from the garnish into a chopper & chop away to your heart's content! I like to go for a fine, liquid-y grind.
• Serve as a dip or a topping for canapés as in picture. I also like to add a tablespoon or so to curries and other Asian stews for a wonderful, tangy depth.
• Store in a sterilized jar for about 2 weeks in the fridge.

Butternut Squash Soup

Ingredients
1. 2 large butternut squashes (peeled, deseeeded and cut into small chunks)
2. 1 large onion (peeled and roughly chopped)

3. 2 vegetable stock cubes
4. 1 potato (about jacket potato size!) peeled and cut into chunks
5. 750ml boiling water (this can be changed depending how thick you like it)
6. 1 tsp Everyday seasoning

Instructions
1. This recipe is very quick and simple because I literally just put it all into a pan and cook for 20-25 mins until all vegetables are tender and then allow to cool (so it doesn't splash and burn!) and then blitz it with a hand blender. I guess you could use a food processor but it's more washing up and I am lazy!

Notes
1. I often use the frozen prepared bags from Morrisons if I am feeling lazy or short of time as they are often a similar price at around £1 a bag and saves the fuss!

Grilled Chicken Souvlaki

Ingredients
• 1 lb. boneless, skinless chicken breasts, cut into 1-in. chunks
• 3 tbsp. olive oil
• 1/2 tsp. coriander
• 1/2 tsp. dried oregano
• Kosher salt and pepper
• 1 pt. grape tomatoes
• 2 cloves garlic, chopped

- 3 tbsp. fresh lemon juice
- 1/2 head romaine lettuce, shredded
- 4 scallions, thinly sliced
- 1/2 c. fresh dill, roughly chopped
- 4 pieces pita bread
- Low-fat Greek yogurt, for serving
- 8 skewers

Directions
1. Heat grill to medium-high. In a large bowl, toss chicken with 1 Tbsp oil, then coriander, oregano, and 1/4 tsp each salt and pepper. Thread onto skewers.
2. Place tomatoes and garlic on a large piece of heavy-duty foil. Drizzle with 1 Tbsp oil and sprinkle with 1/4 tsp each salt and pepper. Fold and seal the foil to form a pouch.
3. Place pouch and skewers on the grill and cook, shaking the pouch and turning kebabs occasionally, until chicken is cooked through, 8 to 10 minutes. Just before removing from the grill, brush chicken with 1 Tbsp lemon juice.
4. Meanwhile, in a large bowl, toss lettuce, scallions, and dill with remaining 2 Tbsp lemon juice and Tbsp oil, plus pinch each salt and pepper. If desired, grill pita bread until warm, about 1 minute per side.
5. Spread pita with yogurt if desired, then stuff with chicken, tomatoes, and salad.

Chickpea-less Beet Hummus (oil-free)

Ingredients
- 1 cup cauliflower florets, steamed
- 3 small cooked beets (roasted or steamed)

- 2 garlic cloves
- 1/3 cup tahini
- 1/3 cup raw walnuts
- Juice from 1/2 lemon
- 1 bag of Harvest Snap Snapea Crisps

Instructions
- In a food processor combine all ingredients (except the Harvest Snaps)
- Keep pulsing until ingredients are blended together and creamy (if it isn't getting creamy, add more tahini)
- Enjoy with Harvest Snaps Snappea Crisps, Lentil Bean or Black Bean snacks!
- Beet hummus will stay good in fridge for 5 days

Healthy Fried Rice Recipe

Ingredients
- 1 tablespoon avocado oil (or other healthy cooking oil), divided
- 3 large eggs
- 5–6 scallions (aka green onions), root and 2 inches of green top removed, chopped (about 1/2 cup)
- 1 large carrot, shredded or julienned (about 1/2 cup)
- 1/2 cup frozen peas
- 2 cups cooked brown rice*
- 3 tablespoons organic tamari** or low sodium soy sauce
- 1 teaspoon rice vinegar (no sugar added)
- 1 teaspoon toasted sesame oil
- 1/2 teaspoon freshly grated ginger
- big pinch of sea salt (more or less to taste)

• a few spins freshly ground black pepper

Instructions
1. Heat 1/2 tablespoon oil over medium heat.
2. In a mixing bowl, whisk the eggs into a uniform mixture until well combine and season with a small pinch of sea salt and fresh black pepper.
3. Add the eggs to the pan and scramble. Once cooked remove the scrambled eggs from the pan to a plate and reserve for later.
4. Add the remaining 1/2 tablespoon oil to the pan over medium heat; add the scallions and carrot and sauté 3-4 minutes until softened.
5. Add the frozen peas to the pan, then add the rice, tamari, rice vinegar, toasted sesame oil and ginger. Stir well to combine, the heat from the pan will quickly defrost the peas.
6. Turn off the heat and stir in the scrambled eggs. Season with a pinch of sea salt if needed–it will depend on the sodium content of the tamari and other ingredients.
7. Turn the heat to low and cook another 5 minutes until the entire dish is warmed through.
8. Water chestnuts, bean sprouts, edamame, just about any other veggie you like, or plain shredded chicken would also be a delicious addition to this dish.

Notes
1. Grab some cooked brown rice on the hot bar at the store to make this even easier. Frozen brown rice also works, defrost it first. Or, cook your rice from scratch according to the package instructions. Any white rice can also be substituted if you prefer.

2. Tamari is gluten-free soy sauce and tastes just like regular soy sauce. You can find it in the ethnic aisle of most grocery stores or at an Asian market. Substitute low-sodium soy sauce if desired.

Rustic Tomato Soup

Ingredients
Makes 2 Servings
• 1/2 yellow onion, diced
• 2 cloves garlic, minced
• 4 Roma tomatoes, chopped
• 1/4 bunch or 1 tsp (5 mL) fresh thyme
• 1/4 tsp (1.2 mL) iodized salt
• 1/4 tsp (1.2 mL) ground black pepper
• 1/8 tsp (0.6 mL) ground cumin
• 1/2 c (95 g) brown rice
• 1/4 tsp (1.2 mL) crushed red pepper (optional)
Directions
1. Saute the onion over medium heat until it just starts to brown. Add the garlic, sauteing for another minute.
2. Add 1 c (240 mL) of water and the remaining ingredients (including optional crushed red pepper if desired), except for the rice. Simmer until tomatoes are soft. Smash the tomatoes with your spoon as they cook until they have turned into sauce.
3. Add the rice and cover the pot. Reduce the heat to low and cook for 25 minutes. If you would like to add a cup of rinsed, red beans to this dish you can do so once the soup is removed from the heat.

4. Note: Use a short-grain brown rice in this dish for a chewier texture.

Noom Friendly Instant Pot Split Lentil Soup

Ingredients
4 servings
• 1 cup washed split red lentil
• 1/2 cup washed brown rice
• 2 diced red onion
• 1 diced carrot
• 4 cups chicken broth
• 2 cup water
• 1 teaspoon salt and pepper
• 1 tablespoon cumin
• 1 teaspoon garlic powder
• 1 teaspoon turmeric
• 1/2 teaspoon ground ginger
• 2 tablespoon olive oil

Cooking Instructions
• Add everything to the Instant Pot and stir. Remember to wash the lentils and rice. A good trick to having the Instant Pot start cooking faster is to boil the water in a kettle beforehand.
• Set the Instant Pot to cook on high for 30 minutes. Let it cool naturally. Stir and serve.

Healthy Jambalaya (Whole30, Low Carb, Paleo)

Ingredients
• 1 pound sausage like Aidell's chicken-apple sausage for Whole30, sliced
• 1 ½ tablespoons olive oil or avocado oil
• 4 cloves garlic minced
• 1 red bell pepper deseeded and chopped (about 1 ½ cups)
• 1 green bell pepper deseeded and chopped (about 1 ½ cups)
• 1 stick celery thinly sliced
• ½ of one onion chopped
• 1 ½ – 2 tablespoons Cajun seasoning
• 1 teaspoon black pepper
• ½ – 1 ½ teaspoons salt use ½ teaspoon if your Cajun seasoning contains salt, up to 1 ½ teaspoons if it doesn't
• ⅛ teaspoon cayenne pepper optional
• 2 14.5-ounce cans fire-roasted tomatoes 29 ounces total
• 1 cup chicken broth
• 5 cups frozen cauliflower rice
• 1 pound medium raw shrimp peeled
• green onions sliced, for garnish
• fresh parsley chopped, for garnish
• Louisiana hot sauce to serve, optional

Instructions
• In a large heavy-bottomed pot or Dutch oven, heat ½ tablespoon olive or avocado oil over medium heat. Add sliced sausage and cook until browned on both sides, stirring occasionally. Transfer sausage to a plate.
• Add 1 tablespoon oil. Add garlic, onion, bell pepper, and celery; sauté until softened, about 5-7 minutes over medium heat.

• Add Cajun seasoning, starting with 1 ½ tablespoons, black pepper, salt, and optional cayenne pepper to pot; stir. Add tomatoes, chicken broth, and sausage to pot, and stir to mix.
• Bring mixture to a boil then reduce heat to low; simmer for 25-35 minutes or until thickened and liquid is reduced.
• Stir in shrimp and cauliflower rice. Cook on low, stirring regularly until rice is heated through and shrimp turn pink and no longer translucent. Don't overcook the shrimp.
• Ladle into bowls and top with sliced green onions and parsley. Serve with Louisiana hot sauce.

Oil-Free Hummus

INGREDIENTS
• 3 cups cooked chickpeas (garbanzo beans) - (cooked in a crock-pot or in an Instant Pot)
• 3 - 6 cloves garlic
• 3/4 cup (approximately) liquid from cooking the chickpeas
• 3 tablespoons roasted tahini - more or less to taste
• 1/4 cup + 2 teaspoons lemon juice
• 1/2 teaspoon granulated onion
• 1/4 teaspoon cumin
• 1 teaspoon salt

Optional Garnishes
• chopped fresh parsley, minced garlic, and/or paprika

INSTRUCTIONS
1. Drain chickpeas, reserving liquid.

2. Place all ingredients in blender and blend until smooth, using as much chickpea liquid as needed to achieve desired consistency. Note: I find this blends best if blended on low speed.
3. Garnish if desired.

Banana Cookie Overnight Oats

Ingredients
• 1 1/2 Cup Old Fashioned Oats
• 1 1/2 Cup Unsweetened Almond Milk
• 1 Cup Non-Fat Greek Yogurt
• 2 Whole Ripe Bananas
• 1 Teaspoon Cinnamon
• 3 Tablespoons Chia Seeds (Optional if you want a completely Green-Zone Breakfast)

Directions
• Mash up the two bananas in a bowl and add all the other ingredients together.
• Stir well and transfer to a mason jar or a cup with a lid.
• Place in the refrigerator overnight.
• In the morning, add any toppings like walnuts, bananas, cinnamon, or blueberries.

LEMON GARLIC SHRIMP PASTA

Ingredients
FOR THE SHRIMP
• 2 lbs shrimp, peeled and deveined

• 1 tbsp minced garlic (about 2 large cloves)
• 1 tsp olive oil
• 1/4 tsp red pepper flakes
• 1/2 tsp kosher salt
FOR THE PASTA
• 8 oz whole wheat or bean-based spaghetti, like Banza chickpea pasta
• 8 oz asparagus, chopped into bite-sized pieces
• 1 tsp olive oil
• 1 tbsp minced garlic
• 1 tsp italian seasoning
• 1/4 tsp kosher salt
• 1 lemon, cut in half
• 4 tbsp light butter (see recipe notes)
• cracked black pepper, to taste
• 1/2 cup grated parmesan cheese
• 1/4 cup parsley, chopped (optional)
• 1/2 cup reserved pasta water

Instructions
• In a medium-sized bowl, toss shrimp with 1 tsp olive oil, 1 tbsp minced garlic, 1/2 tsp kosher salt, and 1/4 tsp red pepper flakes. Increase the pepper flakes to 1/2 tsp if you like things spicy. Cover and refrigerate for about 10 minutes.
• Boil pasta in salted water according to package direction, under cooking by about a minute. Reserve 1/2 cup of cooking water. Drain and set aside.
• Coat a very large skillet in cooking spray. Saute shrimp over medium-high heat until just cooked through, about a minute or two a side depending on the size of your shrimp. Transfer cooked shrimp to a bowl and squeeze the juice of 1/2 a lemon over them. Set aside.

• Lower the heat in the same skillet to medium and add in 1 tsp olive oil. Add asparagus to the skillet along with 1 tsp italian seasoning, 1 tbsp minced garlic, and 1/4 tsp salt. Saute until just softened, about 5 minutes. If the browned bits on on the bottom on the skillet start to get too dark, add in a few splashes of reserved pasta water to scrape them up.
• When asparagus is done, lower the heat and add pasta, shrimp, juice of the other half of the lemon, light butter, parmesan cheese, and cracked black pepper. Toss together, adding in pasta water as needed to loosen the sauce.
• Taste for seasoning. Since there is salt in the pasta water, you probably won't need to add more. Garnish with parsley (optional).

Healthy Chicken and Broccoli Stir Fry

Ingredients
• 1 pound chicken thighs, cut into small pieces
• 4 cloves garlic, minced
• 1 tsp ginger, minced
• 1 tsp salt
• ¼ tsp black pepper
• 1 tsp red pepper flakes
• 1 tbsp avocado oil
• 4 cups broccoli florets
• ⅓ cup water
• ¼ cup coconut aminos
• 1 tsp fish sauce
• 1 ½ tsp sesame oil
• ½ tbsp arrowroot starch
• Green onion, for garnish
• Sesame seeds, for garnish

Method
1. Add the chicken thighs, garlic, ginger, salt, black pepper, and red pepper flakes to a small bowl and stir until well combined.
2. Heat a large skillet over medium-high heat. Once hot, coat the pan with oil and then add in the chicken. Cook the chicken for 6-8 minutes until browned and cooked through. Once cooked, remove the chicken from pan and set aside.
3. While the chicken is cooking, make the sauce. Add the coconut aminos, fish sauce, sesame oil and arrowroot starch to a small bowl and whisk until well combined.
4. Next, add in the broccoli florets and ⅓ cup of water. Cook the broccoli until it is bright green and slightly tender, around 4-6 minutes.
5. Next, add the chicken back to the skillet and then add the sauce. Give everything a stir to combine chicken, broccoli, and sauce are all well combined and cook for one more minute. The sauce should thicken a bit as it heats.
6. Remove the skillet from the heat, finish with sliced green onions and sesame seeds, and then serve the stir-fry immediately. Enjoy!

Quick and easy ratatouille recipe

Ingredients
1. 2 onions, diced
2. 1 aubergine, cut into bite size cubes
3. 2 large courgettes cut into bite size pieces
4. 1 large red pepper cut into bite size pieces
5. 1 large yellow pepper cut into bite sized pieces
6. 2 cloves of garlic, crushed
7. 400g can of chopped tomatoes

8. 2 tbsp chopped basil (halve if using dried rather than fresh)
9. 2 tbsp chopped parsley (halve if using dried rather than fresh)
10. low-calorie cooking spray

Instructions
1. Using a large saucepan and a good few sprays of the low-calorie cooking spray heat add the courgettes, onions, aubergine, peppers, garlic and cook on a high heat, stirring continuously so they do not stick for 3 minutes.
2. Add the tomatoes and stir well.
3. Reduce the heat and cover the pan then simmer for 15 minutes until all the vegetables are cooked.
4. Remove from the heat and stir through the fresh parsley and basil before serving.

THE BEST HUMMUS RECIPE (IN 3 MINUTES!)

INGREDIENTS
• 2 (15-ounce cans) chickpeas, drained with liquid reserved
• ⅓ cup chickpea liquid, or more, as needed
• ½ cup tahini
• ¼ cup olive oil
• 2 lemons, juiced
• 2 garlic cloves
• 1 teaspoon cumin
• ½ teaspoon kosher salt
FOR GARNISH
• extra-virgin olive oil
• paprika

• freshly chopped parsley

INSTRUCTIONS

1. Add all the ingredients to a high-powered blender and secure the lid. Remove the lid cap and insert the tamper.

2. Turn the blender on high for 30 seconds (or more for a creamier texture) and use the tamper to push the hummus into the blades. Add more chickpea liquid (aquafaba), if desired, for a softer hummus.

3. Add the hummus to a small serving bowl and garnish with olive oil, paprika and fresh parsley.

LISA'S TIPS
• Don't forget that you can also make tahini yourself (rather than buying in the store). Just follow my tahini recipe.
• The Vitamix blender I use is the Vitamix Ascent 3500 – and I love it!
• 1 cup of dried chickpeas = 3 cups of soaked and cooked chickpeas = approx 30 ounces canned chickpeas

Curried Cauliflower Soup

Equipment
• Immersion Blender
• Large pot

Ingredients

- 1 tablespoon extra-virgin olive oil or coconut oil
- 1 large yellow onion quartered and sliced
- 1 tablespoon curry powder see notes
- 4 cups vegetable broth or chicken broth
- 1 teaspoon kosher salt plus more to taste
- 1 head cauliflower cut into florets (about 24 oz.)
- 2 medium zucchini grated
- lime wedges, fresh cilantro, extra cauliflower and zucchini, plain yogurt, sunflower seeds, etc. for garnish, optional

Instructions

- In a large pot, sauté the sliced onion in the olive oil (1 tablespoon) and the curry powder (1 tablespoon) over medium heat until onions are softened and curry power is fragrant.
- Add the vegetable broth (4 cups), the cauliflower florets, and the kosher salt (1 teaspoon). Bring to a boil, cover, and simmer on low for about 15 minutes, or until cauliflower is tender.
- Use an immersion blender to puree the soup to desired consistency (or a standing blender in batches). Stir in the grated zucchini and simmer for 3-5 more minutes, until zucchini is softened a bit.
- Taste and adjust seasoning as necessary. Serve with extra veggies, a squeeze of fresh lime juice, and a garnish of fresh cilantro, if desired.

Notes

- Boost the flavor: this recipe is simple and minimalist, but delicious. But for an extra boost of flavor, try adding some minced garlic and fresh ginger with the onions. You can also add a can of coconut milk in place of 1 cup of the broth for a richer, creamier consistency.

• For an extra-smooth consistency, omit the grated zucchini.

• Curry powders vary greatly in type and spice level, so you may need to use more or less than 1 tablespoon. If you aren't familiar with the curry powder you are using, start with 1 teaspoon and add more if needed after pureeing the soup.

• Store in your fridge in an airtight container for up to 5 days. Freeze for up to 6 months.

• Recipe adapted from "Curried Cauliflower Soup" on Noom's recipe database.

15-Minute Spinach Tomato Frittata

Ingredients

1 tbsp Extra virgin olive oil
2 stalk(s) Green onion (thinly sliced)
1 bag(s) Baby spinach
3 large egg Egg
5 large egg Egg white
1 tbsp Extra virgin olive oil
1 cup Cherry Tomatoes
4 slice Mozzarella cheese, partially skimmed
4 slice Whole grain bread (toasted)
Instructions
1. Preheat broiler.
2. Heat olive oil in large ovenproof nonstick skillet over medium heat. Cook scallions 1 minute, stirring, or until softened.

3. Transfer scallions to large bowl and set aside. Add spinach, whole eggs, and egg whites to the bowl with the scallions. Beat with fork until well blended.

4. Heat remaining oil in skillet over medium heat. Pour in egg mixture and scatter tomatoes on top. Cover skillet and cook 4 minutes, or until eggs are set around edges.

5. Broil 5" from heat 4 minutes, or until frittata is lightly browned and the center is set. Top with cheese, cover, and let stand 1 minute to melt cheese. Cut into 4 wedges and serve.

Healthy low-calorie Shakshuka recipe

Ingredients
1. 800g chopped tomatoes (2 x 400g tins if you are in UK)
2. 2 large red peppers
3. 4 cloves of garlic finally chopped
4. 1 large brown onion
5. 4 large fresh eggs
6. 2 tbsp of tomato puree
7. 1 tsp smoked paprika
8. 1 tsp ground cumin
9. 1 tsp of chilli powder (if using)
10. 1/2 tsp sea salt
11. 2 tbsp of fresh herb of choice
12. 2 tbsp of olive oil

Instructions
1. Preheat your oven to 180°c
2. In a large ovenproof deep pan or skillet, slowly warm up your oil and gently sauté the onions and peppers for 5 minutes.

3. When they have softened slightly, add the garlic, tomato puree and spices and mix together on a low heat. Frying the spices this way releases all the fragrance and aroma.
4. After 2 minutes add in your chopped tomatoes and half of the fresh herbs, let it all simmer together for 5 minutes on a low heat. Season with salt, and taste.
5. Using the back of a spoon, make 4 wells, spaced apart for your eggs to be placed. Gently crack in each egg being careful not to burst the yolk!

Vegetable and Chickpea Paella

Ingredients
1. 250g Paella rice (dried)
2. 1.5 litres vegetable stock
3. 3 cloves garlic crushed
4. 1 400g can Chickpeas (drained)
5. 2 tbsp. smoked paprika
6. 1 tbsp. Turmeric
7. 4 peppers deseeded and cut into small chunks
8. 2 small red onions peeled and finely chopped
9. 3 small red onions peeled and quartered
10. Large handful of baby spinach
11. 15 cherry tomatoes halved
12. 200g Mushrooms (sliced)
13. Low-Calorie cooking spray

Instructions
1. Using low-calorie cooking spray in a large frying pan placed over medium-high heat, fry garlic and the chopped onion until soft.

2. Add paella rice and fry gently for 2 minutes.
3. Add two ladles of stock and stir gently until the rice has absorbed all the liquid.
4. Add the remainder of the stock and cook for 10 minutes still on medium-high heat.
5. Add paprika, turmeric, quartered onions, peppers, chickpeas and mushrooms and turn heat to medium.
6. Cook for a further 5 minutes then add halved cherry tomatoes and cook for a further 5 minutes.
7. Add the spinach and stir through. As soon as the spinach has wilted a little serve immediately.

Balsamic Honey Chicken

Ingredients
• 4 boneless, skinless chicken breast halves
• salt
• ground black pepper
• 1 tbsp. extra-virgin olive oil
• 2 cloves garlic, chopped
• 2 medium bosc pears, peeled, cored, and sliced
• 1 c. reduced-sodium chicken broth
• 1/4 c. balsamic vinegar
• 1 1/2 tbsp. honey
• 1 1/2 tsp. cornstarch

Directions
1. Rinse the chicken in cold water. Then pat dry with paper towels. Place each chicken breast half between two sheets of plastic wrap and pound the chicken breasts to 1/2" thick.

Remove the plastic and sprinkle both sides of each breast with salt and pepper to taste.

2. In a large skillet over medium-high heat, heat the oil. Add the chicken and cook for 3 to 4 minutes on each side, turning once, until it's no longer pink in the center and the juices run clear. Remove the chicken from the heat and transfer it to a platter. Cover it to keep it warm.

3. Add the garlic and turn the heat down to medium for 2 minutes, or until the garlic is soft. Add the pears and continue cooking for 3 to 4 minutes, stirring occasionally, until the pears are soft and golden brown.

4. In a small bowl, combine the chicken broth, balsamic vinegar, honey, and cornstarch. Pour over the pear mixture. Increase the heat to high until it comes to a boil, and then immediately lower the heat and simmer, stirring frequently for 4 to 6 minutes, or until the sauce thickens slightly. Return the chicken and any juices to the pan and cook for 1 to 2 minutes. Taste and adjust the seasoning, if necessary.

5. Place the chicken on individual serving plates or on a large platter. Use a slotted spoon to mound the fruit over the top. Spoon the sauce over the fruit and around the chicken. Serve immediately.

Prik Noom Recipe (Northern Thai Green Chili Dip)

INGREDIENTS
• 5-6 long green chili peppers
• 6 garlic cloves
• 4 Thai shallots or 2 normal shallots
• 1-2 teaspoons lime juice
• 1/2 teaspoon palm sugar white sugar or brown are also ok

• 2-3 sprigs fresh coriander
• 1-2 tablespoons fish sauce

INSTRUCTIONS
1. Add chilis, garlic, and shallots to a pan over a medium heat.
2. Leave the ingredients in the pan long enough so that they become scorched. Don't worry about blackened skin: we will be discarding this.
3. Remove ingredients from the heat and leave to cool for five minutes. After five minutes, peel the skins from the shallots, chilis, and garlic. The skins should peel off easily.
4. Place chilis, shallots, and garlic in a mortar. Pound the ingredients together until they form a coarse consistency and they are thoroughly mixed.
5. Add fish sauce, sugar, lime juice, and pound a couple more times. Serve in a small bowl and dip fried meet, boiled vegetables, or sticky rice into the nam prik noom. Enjoy one of Northern Thailand's tastiest treats!

Raspberry Lime Smoothie from Noom

INGREDIENTS
• 2 cups hulled raspberries, blueberries, or strawberries
• 1 banana
• 1/2 cup orange juice
• 1 tbsp lime
• 1/2 cup crushed ice
• 2 mint leaves or lime wedges garnish

INSTRUCTIONS
• Combine all the ingredients in a blender (except garnish) and blund until smooth
• Pour into 2 glasses and garnish with mint leaves or lime wedge

STRAWBERRY BANANA SMOOTHIE

INGREDIENTS
• 1 cup frozen strawberries
• 1 frozen banana , cut into pieces
• 1 cup milk (I use almond milk)
• 1/2 cup orange juice (or use more milk)
• 1 Medjool date , pitted (or 1 tablespoon honey), if needed for sweetness

INSTRUCTIONS

• Add the strawberries, banana, milk, orange juice, and date for sweetness, if desired, and blend until smooth. Taste and adjust anything as needed, then serve right away.
• Leftover smoothie can be poured into mini ice pop molds for a frozen treat later.

Green Monster Smoothie

Ingredients
• 1 cup plain or vanilla coconut milk, I use Silk Brand PureCoconut
• 6-8 oz vanilla greek yogurt
• 1 RIPE, frozen banana
• 2-4 cups raw, organic spinach (I use 3 cups)

Instructions
• Place all ingredients into a blender.
• Blend & liquify
• Serve

Wake-Up Smoothie

Ingredients
• 1 ¼ cups orange juice, preferably calcium-fortified
• 1 banana
• 1 ¼ cups frozen berries, such as raspberries, blackberries, blueberries and/or strawberries
• 1/2 cup low-fat silken tofu, or low-fat plain yogurt
• 1 tablespoon sugar, or Splenda Granular (optional)

Directions
1. Combine orange juice, banana, berries, tofu (or yogurt) and sugar (or Splenda), if using, in a blender; cover and blend until creamy. Serve immediately.

Our Favorite Berry Smoothie

Ingredients
• ½ cup vanilla yogurt
• 2 cups mixed berries frozen
• 1 tablespoon chia seeds
• 1 cup milk

Instructions
• Add yogurt, berries, chia seeds and milk to blender.
• Blend until smooth.
• Serve immediately.

Healthy Coffee Smoothie Recipe

EQUIPMENT
• Vitamix

INGREDIENTS
• 1 tablespoon ground coffee un-brewed, (not instant coffee)
• 1 tablespoon peanut butter

• ½ teaspoon vanilla extract
• ¾ cup unsweetened almond milk (or milk of choice)
• ¼ cup brewed coffee, chilled (Try my organic coffee beans)
• ½ frozen banana (the riper, the sweeter)
• raw honey, as needed, for sweetness (and if not vegan)
• ice, as needed to thicken

INSTRUCTIONS
To Make the Healthy Coffee Smoothie Recipe:
• Add all the ingredients to a blender and blend until smooth.
• Add more ice if too liquidy or more almond milk if too thick, as needed.
• Serve immediately.
To Make The Smoothie Freezer Pack:
• To make the smoothie freezer pack, add the ground coffee to the bottom of the bag, followed by banana, vanilla extract, and peanut butter to a freezer bag.
• Press the air out of the bag and seal tightly, then place in the freezer.
• When ready to blend, add the almond milk and chilled coffee to a blender, followed by the frozen contents from the freezer pack.
• Blend until smooth.

Pumpkin Smoothie

Ingredients
• 1/2 cup pumpkin puree
• 1/2 cup milk of choice

• 1/2 cup crushed ice
• 6 oz nonfat Greek or plain yogurt
• 2 tsp vanilla extract
• 1/2 tsp pumpkin pie spice or cinnamon, or more to taste
• 2 tsp packed brown sugar, or maple syrup to taste
• add a scoop of vanilla protein, optional

Instructions
• Put all ingredients in a blender and blend until smooth. Divide in two cups.
• Serve with a straw.

Cranberry smoothie

Ingredients
1. 500ml Ocean Spray Cranberry Juice
2. 1 Peeled and sliced banana
3. 1 apple, washed, cored and cut into wedges
4. 75g mixed frozen berries such as strawberries, blueberries or mixed berries

Instructions
1. Pour the cranberry juice into a blender and then add the berries, banana and apple.
2. Whizz on high power until all combined well and the smoothie becomes a perfect velvet-like texture.
3. Serve immediately

Healthy Overnight Oats For Weight Loss (Vegan)

EQUIPMENT
• 1 small jar with a lid
• 1 Spoon

INGREDIENTS
• ½ cup rolled/old fashioned oats
• ½ cup oat milk
• 1 tablespoon chia seeds
• 1 tablespoon pure maple syrup
• ⅓ cup mixed fresh/frozen fruit of choice optional

INSTRUCTIONS
• In a small jar or airtight container, mix rolled oats, chia seeds, maple syrup, and oat milk (or your favorite dairy-free milk). Stir all the ingredients together until the oats are completely covered. Cover the jar with a lid.
• Transfer the jar to the fridge and let the oats soak overnight.
• In the morning, stir the oats again and if the mixture is too dense add a few splashes of milk. Top it with fresh/frozen fruit of choice, nuts, or seeds you love. Drizzle with maple syrup or peanut butter to make it sweeter. Dig in and enjoy!

NOTES
• Use only plain (sugar-free) rolled oats without any artificial flavors
• Fruit, seeds, and nut butter of choice can be added while you prepare the oats, before storing them in the fridge
• If you more ingredients add enough milk to completely soak the oats

• If you need a bigger batch simply double or triple the recipe ingredients and use a bigger container
• It's best to let the oats soak overnight but if you are short on time you can soak them for at least 2 hours
Nutrition facts for 1 serving are calculated without the additional toppings

Weight Loss Soup

EQUIPMENT
• Crock Pot (Slow Cooker)

INGREDIENTS
• 32 ounces chicken broth you may use low-sodium
• 3 cups V-8 juice *see recipe notes
• 28 ounces Italian diced tomatoes
• 1 small onion
• 2 cloves minced garlic
• 8 ounces sliced mushrooms
• 3 carrots peeled and sliced
• 1 zucchini diced
• 1 yellow squash diced
• 2 cups green beans fresh or frozen
• 14 ounces kidney beans drained and rinsed
• 3 to 4 cups shredded cabbage
• 1 teaspoons Italian seasoning
• salt and pepper

INSTRUCTIONS

• In a large frying pan sprayed with cooking spray, saute garlic, onions, carrots, and mushrooms for about 5 minutes.
• In a large crockpot, combine sauteed garlic and vegetables with the remaining ingredients.
• Cook on high for 2-3 hours, or until vegetables are fork-tender.

FREEZING INSTRUCTIONS
1. This makes a large batch of soup. If you would like to freeze portions of it to use later, undercook the vegetables just a little. Pour the soup into freezer Ziplock bags and let as much air out as you can. Lay the bags flat on a cookie sheet and freeze. Once the soup is frozen flat, it is easy to layer in your freezer and won't take up much room. To thaw, place the bag in the fridge for 24 hours and then reheat.

Vegetable Skillet Frittata from NOOM

INGREDIENTS
• 1 cup low-fat cottage cheese
• 2 eggs
• 4 egg whites
• ¼ cup chicken broth reduced sodium
• 1 cup chopped onions
• 1 cup sliced green beans
• 1 cup chopped broccoli
• ¼ cup shredded carrot
• 2 cloves garlic minced
• ½ tsp ground black pepper
• ¼ tsp salt

• ⅓ cup shredded sharp cheddar cheese reduced-fat

INSTRUCTIONS
• Combine the cottage cheese, eggs, and egg whites in a blender or food processor. Pulse until very smooth. Set aside
• Bring the broth and onions to a boil in a large nonstick skillet over medium heat. Cook for 5 minutes or until onions soften
• Add the beans, broccoli, carrot, and garlic. Cover and continue cooking for 2 minutes or until broccoli is bright green
• Season with salt and pepper. Add the egg mixture and cheese.
• Reduce heat to low, cover and cook for 15 minutes or until eggs are set
• Cut into wedges and serve

Easy Healthy Banana Oat Waffles

Ingredients
• 1 cup rolled oats
• 2 medium bananas chopped
• 2 eggs
• 1 teaspoon vanilla extract
• 1 teaspoon baking powder
• pinch of salt optional
• to serve
• Fresh fruit of your choice
• honey/maple syrup
• peanut/almond butter
• yoghurt

Instructions
• Place all the batter ingredients in a blender and blend until smooth.
• Heat a waffle maker/iron then spray with non-stick cooking spray. Pour in a few tablespoons of batter.
• Cook until the waffles are golden brown and cooked through.
• Carefully remove the waffles and serve with toppings of your choice.

TROPICAL RASPBERRY SMOOTHIE

INGREDIENTS
• 1 cup water or milk of choice
• 1 cup frozen raspberries
• 1 banana
• 2 tablespoons lime juice
• 1 teaspoon coconut oil
• 1 teaspoon agave
• Ice

INSTRUCTIONS
1. Blend all ingredients in a high-speed blender until smooth. Add ice, if desired

LOW CALORIE PEANUT BUTTER BANANA SMOOTHIE

INGREDIENTS
• ¼ Cup (60mL) Unsweetened Vanilla Almond Milk

• 1 Banana (100g)
• ⅔ Cup (66g) Powdered Peanut Butter
• 1 Tbsp (12g) Sugar Substitute
• 1 ½ Cups of ice (200g)
• Pinch of Salt

INSTRUCTIONS
1. Add all ingredients into your blender and blend until smooth

Chocolate Chia Seed Pudding

INGREDIENTS
• 1/4 cup unsweetened cocoa powder
• 1/2 cup hot brewed coffee
• 1/4 cup chia seeds
• 3/4 cup plain, unsweetened soy milk (or any plant-based milk)
• 2 tablespoons maple syrup
• 1 pinch sea salt

INSTRUCTIONS
• Add the cocoa powder and hot coffee to a small mixing bowl and whisk well. Add the rest of the ingredients to and whisk well to combine. Place in the fridge for 1-2 hours until firm or overnight. Try to whisk again in the first 5-10 minutes of chilling as some clumps may form.

NOTES

• Chilling time: Although it's easiest to chill the chia pudding overnight, I find that it usually set within a couple of hours of chilling (about 2 hours).
• For smooth texture: Don't like the lumpy texture of chia pudding? Simply add your chia pudding to a blender before chilling and puree until smooth. This recipe blends best in a single serving smoothie cup. For best results, double or triple the recipe is you want to blend in your smoothie pitcher.
• Topping suggestions: fresh fruit, granola, chopped nuts, nut butter, cocoa nibs, chocolate shavings, coconut chips, crumbled cookies, vegan whipped cream.

Pumpkin Pie Overnight Oats with Chia

Ingredients
• 1/4 cup plain nonfat greek yogurt (or use vanilla!)
• 1/2 cup unsweetened vanilla almond milk (or any milk)
• 1/4 cup pumpkin puree
• 1-2 tablespoons pure maple syrup
• 1/2 teaspoon vanilla extract
• 1/2 cup rolled oats (gluten free if desired)
• 2 teaspoons chia seeds
• 1/2 teaspoon pumpkin pie spice

Instructions
• In a medium bowl, mix together greek yogurt, almond milk, pumpkin puree, vanilla and 1 tablespoon maple syrup until well combined.

• Stir in oats, chia seeds and pumpkin pie spice. Taste and add more maple syrup if you want it sweeter. Pour into a glass jar or container and place in fridge for 4 hours or overnight. Makes 1 serving of pumpkin overnight oats.